GLUCOSE TRANSFORMATION

How Maintaining a Healthy Blood Sugar Level Can Alter Your Life.

By

Ruben M. McDonald

Copyright © by Ruben M. McDonald|2024. All rights reserved.

Dear reader, I make the results of current scientific research understandable to anyone in this book. turn them into useful advice. Keep in mind that none of this is medical advice—I'm a researcher, not a physician.

See your doctor ahead of utilizing any of the tips in this publication if you take any medications or have any health issues.

Glucose Transformation: How Maintaining a Healthy Blood Sugar Level Can Alter Your Life

BE INSPIRED

Success Stories: Actual Persons, Actual Outcomes

Stories of real people succeeding in controlling their blood sugar might serve as an inspiration and source of motivation for those facing comparable obstacles. Here are a few instances of these kinds of triumphs:

John's Path to Diabetes Type 2 Reversal:

After receiving a type 2 diabetes diagnosis, John found it difficult to control his blood sugar levels with medicine alone. He set out on a voyage of lifestyle adjustments, determined to take charge of his health.

He started eating a whole-food, plant-based diet full of fruits, vegetables, legumes, and whole grains. He also started doing weight training and walking regularly.

John experienced gradual improvements in his blood sugar readings, increased levels of fitness, and reduced weight. He was able to reverse his type 2 diabetes with the help of medical professionals, and he is now living a healthier, more active life.

Mike's Transformation through Coaching and Individualized Nutrition: Mike, a middle-aged person with prediabetes, sought assistance from a medical team that specialized in lifestyle modifications and individualized nutrition.

Mike obtained individualized coaching sessions, genetic testing, and biomarker analysis to obtain recommendations for food adjustments, workout regimens, stress reduction strategies, and sleep optimization.

Mike was able to successfully lower his blood sugar levels, enhance his insulin sensitivity, lose excess weight, and lessen his chance of developing type 2 diabetes with several months of committed effort and supervision. With continuous care and observation, he keeps up his health.

Maria's Path to Enhanced Blood Sugar Regulation through Mindfulness:

Maria, a working mother with type 2 diabetes, found it difficult to put her health first in the face of stress and everyday obligations. She learned how effective mindfulness exercises were at controlling her blood sugar.

By implementing mindfulness practices like meditation, breathing exercises, and mindful eating, Maria was able to lower her stress levels, increase her present-moment awareness, and make better decisions.

When regular mindfulness exercises were included in Maria's daily routine, she saw improvements in her emotional health, more stable blood sugar levels, and a stronger sense of control over her diabetes.

These success stories demonstrate the variety of approaches people can use to improve blood sugar control. Through lifestyle changes, technology improvements, individualized treatment plans, or mindfulness exercises, each narrative emphasizes the value of perseverance, knowledge, and support in overcoming obstacles and reaching long-term success in controlling blood sugar levels and general health.

Testimonials and Blood Sugar Balancing Experiences

Linda's Testimonial: "I was resolved to take charge of my health organically and avoid medicine after receiving a prediabetes diagnosis. My healthcare practitioner helped me make little but significant dietary and lifestyle adjustments. I concentrated on eating healthier foods, cutting back on sugar and processed carbohydrates, and exercising frequently by going for walks and doing yoga. My blood sugar levels eventually stabilized, and I also started to lose weight. Maintaining blood sugar balance has enhanced my general well-being, vitality, and health."

Jenny's Path to Mindful Eating: "I've been able to better manage my blood sugar levels and my relationship with food thanks to mindful eating." I take the time to enjoy every bite of food, pay attention to signals of hunger and fullness, and make thoughtful food selections rather than speeding through meals. This method has normalized my blood sugar readings and lessened my cravings for sweet foods. I now eat mindfully every day, which makes me happy and benefits my health and mind."

David's Success with Herbal Supplements: "I chose to look into natural alternatives after years of dealing with insulin resistance and erratic blood sugar levels. I included a balanced diet, frequent exercise, and herbal supplements like bebeerine and cinnamon in my daily routine. I was shocked to see that both my blood sugar and energy levels had returned to normal. I'm happy with the outcomes, and these herbal pills have become a crucial component of my blood sugar management plan."

Anna's Path to Tailored Nutrition: "It has changed my life to work with a registered dietitian to develop a tailored nutrition plan. My meals and snacks have been optimized by knowing which foods are ideal for my body and blood sugar levels. My focus is on mindful portion sizes, well-balanced macronutrients, and nutrient-dense foods. This method has helped me better control my blood sugar levels and has taught me how to feed my body in a way that promotes my general health and vigor."

These testimonies and firsthand accounts demonstrate the variety of strategies people might employ to effectively regulate their blood sugar levels. Personalized nutrition programs, herbal supplements, technology, mindfulness exercises, and dietary modifications are some of the methods used in these stories to emphasize the significance of identifying the most effective approach for specific needs and objectives. It's encouraging to observe how people who prioritize

17 | Page

blood sugar control and general well-being can attain favorable results and enhance their quality of life.

CHAPTER 1

Understanding The Impact of Blood Sugar

As the body's main source of energy for cells, blood sugar, commonly referred to as blood glucose, is essential to bodily functions. For general health and well-being, however, blood sugar regulation is crucial. This section will discuss how blood sugar affects different parts of health and explain why blood sugar regulation is important.

Food, particularly carbs, which are converted into glucose during digestion, is the source of blood sugar. Energy for cellular processes is provided by glucose, which enters the bloodstream and is distributed to all of the body's cells.

Blood Sugar Regulation is Important: There are several reasons why it's important to keep your blood sugar levels at ideal ranges.

Energy Production: A stable supply of energy for cells, tissues, and organs is guaranteed by balanced blood sugar.

Brain Function: The brain uses glucose extensively for memory, cognitive performance, and general mental clarity.

Hormone Regulation: The release of insulin, glucagon, and other hormones related to energy balance and metabolism is influenced by blood sugar levels.

Cellular Health: Overly large blood sugar swings might eventually cause harm to organs, blood vessels, and nerves, which can result in medical issues.

The following are some possible effects of hyperglycemia, or high blood sugar, which can occur when blood sugar levels stay higher for prolonged periods:

Increased Risk of Diabetes: Type 2 diabetes and insulin resistance are linked to persistently elevated blood sugar levels.

Cardiovascular Risk: Heart disease, stroke, and other cardiovascular disorders are made more likely by elevated blood sugar levels.

Elevated blood sugar levels have the potential to harm nerves, resulting in neuropathy and associated issues.

Eyesight and renal Issues: Prolonged hyperglycemia can lead to problems with eyesight and renal function.

Hypoglycemia (Low Blood Sugar): Conversely, hypoglycemia, or low blood sugar, can also have serious consequences.

Energy Slump: Excessive blood sugar levels can lead to weakness, exhaustion, lightheadedness, and trouble focusing.

Anxiety, irritability, mood fluctuations, and hunger pangs can all be caused by hypoglycemia.

Cognitive Impairment: Hypoglycemia that is too severe can cause problems with coordination, cognition, and decision-making. Risk of Complications: Hypoglycemia that is too severe can result in seizures, unconsciousness, and other life-threatening situations.

Blood sugar-related factors include:

The following are some of the elements that affect blood sugar regulation:

Diet: Your blood sugar levels can be influenced by the kinds and quantities of fiber, proteins, fats, and carbohydrates you eat.

Physical Activity: By improving insulin sensitivity and muscle uptake of glucose, exercise helps control blood sugar levels.

Stress: Stress-related chemicals, such as cortisol, can cause swings in blood sugar levels.

Medication: Blood sugar levels can be impacted by several drugs, including

corticosteroids, insulin, and oral
hypoglycemic agents.

It is essential to comprehend the effects
of blood sugar to preserve optimum
health and avoid problems brought on
by abnormal blood sugar levels. People
can support blood sugar regulation and
enhance general well-being by
embracing healthy lifestyle practices,
such as a balanced diet, frequent
exercise, stress management, and
medication adherence for those with
diabetes. Effective blood sugar
management requires strong

collaboration with healthcare providers and routine blood sugar monitoring.

Why It's Important to Maintain Blood Sugar Balance

The preservation of steady blood glucose levels, which is essential for general health and well-being, is referred to as blood sugar balance. Maintaining this equilibrium is crucial for optimum health since the body's capacity to control blood sugar plays a vital role in many physiological processes. We'll look at the importance of blood sugar balance and how it affects several areas of our health in this section.

1. Energy Regulation: Stable blood sugar levels guarantee a constant and reliable flow of energy to all of the body's cells, tissues, and organs. The main energy source for cellular functions and metabolic processes is glucose, which is produced when food's carbs are broken down. 2. Brain Function: The brain is heavily dependent on glucose for energy to sustain cognitive skills including memory, focus, and mental clarity.

2. When blood sugar levels are balanced, energy levels remain consistent, supporting vitality and reducing energy crashes. Maintaining balanced blood sugar levels promotes the best possible brain health by improving mental clarity, focus, and cognitive function. Variations in blood sugar levels can cause weariness, mental fog, and difficulties focusing.

3. Hormonal Balance: The hormones insulin and glucagon, in particular, play a major role in controlling blood sugar levels. While glucagon increases blood sugar levels when they go too low,

insulin helps lower blood sugar levels by promoting glucose uptake into cells. For the regulation of hunger, blood sugar stability, and metabolic health, these hormones must remain in a delicate balance.

4. Weight Management: Metabolic abnormalities and weight gain can be caused by an imbalanced blood sugar level, which is typified by frequent spikes and crashes. Excessive blood sugar levels encourage the production of insulin, which prevents the breakdown of fat and promotes fat storage. Low blood sugar, on the other

hand, can cause overeating and weight gain by causing hunger and desire. To promote good weight management and metabolic function, blood sugar equilibrium must be achieved.

5. Diabetes Prevention and Management: Blood sugar regulation is essential for both preventing and treating diabetes, especially Type 2 diabetes. Long-term high blood sugar, or hyperglycemia, can cause poor glucose tolerance, insulin resistance, and ultimately diabetes. People can lower their chance of acquiring diabetes and improve their management

of the disease if they already have it by adopting lifestyle measures that maintain stable blood sugar levels.

6. Cardiovascular Health: Heart disease, stroke, and hypertension are among the cardiovascular disorders that are linked to elevated blood sugar levels. Endothelial dysfunction, oxidative stress, inflammation, and the development of atherosclerotic plaques in blood arteries are all influenced by persistent hyperglycemia. Maintaining balanced blood sugar levels can lower the risk of consequences from

cardiovascular disease and safeguard cardiovascular health.

7. Consistent Mood and Vitality:

Unbalanced blood sugar levels might affect energy levels and psychological stability. Mood swings, anger, exhaustion, and a decline in mental health might result from rapid blood sugar variations. A more balanced mood, prolonged energy, and an enhanced quality of life can all be supported by maintaining stable blood sugar through balanced nutrition, regular meals, and mindful eating.

A vital component of preserving ideal health and well-being is blood sugar homeostasis. The benefits of normal blood sugar levels are extensive and include everything from hormone balance, weight control, diabetes prevention, energy regulation, brain function, cardiovascular health, and mood stability. People can support blood sugar balance and have better health outcomes by implementing good lifestyle behaviors, such as eating a balanced diet, getting regular exercise, managing their stress, and getting enough sleep. For early detection and treatment, blood sugar levels must be regularly monitored, particularly for those who are at risk of diabetes or metabolic diseases.

The Repercussions of Unbalanced Blood Sugar

A person's general health and well-being can be significantly impacted by blood sugar imbalances, whether they are abnormally low (hypoglycemia) or persistently high (hyperglycemia). Maintaining metabolic balance, energy production, and other physiological processes depend on the body's capacity to control blood sugar. The effects of blood sugar imbalance and their possible effects on various aspects of health will be discussed in this section.

1. Hyperglycemia: The Aftereffects of Elevated Blood Sugar:

a. Elevated Risk of Type 2 Diabetes: Extended hyperglycemia raises the risk of insulin resistance, a condition in which cells lose their sensitivity to the effects of insulin, raising blood sugar levels. This can develop into Type 2 diabetes over time, which is a chronic illness with major health consequences.

b. Cardiovascular Complications: High blood sugar levels have been linked to a higher chance of developing heart disease, stroke, and hypertension, among other cardiovascular disorders. The risk of heart-related issues is increased by chronic hyperglycemia, which also leads to oxidative stress, inflammation, and blood vessel damage.

c. Nerve Damage (Neuropathy): High blood sugar levels can harm nerves all over the body, resulting in neuropathy. Pain, tingling, numbness, and reduced sensation in the extremities are possible symptoms that can limit mobility and quality of life.

d. Eye Issues (Retinopathy): Uncontrolled diabetes and elevated blood sugar levels can cause diabetic retinopathy, which is the resultant damage to blood vessels in the eyes. If treatment for this problem is not received, it may result in blindness, visual loss, and other eye concerns.

a. Kidney Damage (Nephropathy): Diabetic nephropathy is a condition caused by chronic hyperglycemia that damages and impairs the kidneys' blood vessels. If left untreated, this illness can worsen and lead to renal failure.

f. Enhanced Infection Risk: People with high blood sugar have weakened immune systems and poor wound healing, which increases their risk of infection, particularly oral, urinary tract, and skin infections.

Hypoglycemia: The Repercussions of Low Blood Sugar:

a. Energy Slumps: Severe weariness, weakness, and trouble concentrating can result from low blood sugar levels. Daily tasks, output, and cognitive performance may all be impacted by this.

b. Anxiety and Mood Swings: Hypoglycemia can result in agitation, anxiety, irritability, and mood swings. Emotional ups and downs can impact relationships and general well-being.

c. Impaired Cognitive Function: Brain fog, disorientation, and difficulty making decisions can result from severe hypoglycemia's effects on memory, concentration, and cognitive function.

d. Danger of fainting and accidents: Severe hypoglycemia can cause dizziness, lightheadedness, and episodes of fainting. There is a chance for mishaps, falls, and injuries from this, particularly for senior citizens.

b. Confusion and Loss of Consciousness: Severe hypoglycemia can result in convulsions, unconsciousness, and medical emergencies that need quick attention.

The long-term effects of blood sugar imbalances can include impaired general health and a lower quality of life. Both hyperglycemia and hypoglycemia can have these effects if they are not managed or treated. These might consist of:

a. Chronic Health concerns: Several chronic health concerns linked to unbalanced blood sugar levels include diabetes, cardiovascular ailments, nerve damage, eye complications, and renal disorders.

b. Decreased Quality of Life: Chronic blood sugar abnormalities can hurt self-sufficiency, mobility, independence, and day-to-day functioning.

c. Effects on Mental Health: Variations in blood sugar levels over time may contribute to mood disorders, anxiety, depression, and cognitive decline. d. Pregnancy-Related Complications: Unbalanced blood sugar levels during pregnancy (known as gestational diabetes) may result in birth defects, macrosomia (a large birth weight), and delivery complications for both the mother and the unborn child.

Excessive or insufficient blood sugar levels can have detrimental effects on one's health and overall wellness. It's critical to routinely check blood sugar levels, develop healthy lifestyle practices, heed medical advice for managing diabetes or other blood sugar issues, and get help right away if you experience any worrisome symptoms associated with blood sugar imbalances. People can lower their risk of problems and achieve better overall health outcomes by making blood sugar control a priority.

CHAPTER 2

Risks and Health Implications of High Blood Sugar

High blood sugar, commonly known as hyperglycemia, happens when there is an excess of glucose in the bloodstream. Prolonged durations of increased blood sugar can have substantial health repercussions and raise the risk of different problems. In this section, we'll investigate the hazards and health concerns connected with high blood sugar levels.

Increased Risk of Type 2 Diabetes:
High blood sugar is a marker of insulin
resistance and poor glucose
metabolism, both of which are
precursors to Type 2 diabetes. Chronic
hyperglycemia can lead to beta cell
malfunction in the pancreas, lowering
insulin production and worsening blood
sugar abnormalities.

Cardiovascular Complications: a. Heart
Disease: Elevated blood sugar levels
contribute to atherosclerosis (hardening
of arteries) and plaque development,

increasing the risk of coronary artery disease, heart attacks, and angina.

b. Stroke: High blood sugar is a risk factor for ischemic strokes, where the blood supply to the brain is stopped due to narrowed or clogged blood vessels.

c. Hypertension: Chronic hyperglycemia can lead to high blood pressure, further stressing the cardiovascular system and raising the risk of heart disease and stroke.

Nerve Damage (Neuropathy): Prolonged high blood sugar can damage nerves throughout the body,

leading to diabetic neuropathy.
Symptoms may include numbness,
tingling, discomfort, and diminished
sensation in the extremities.
Neuropathy can compromise mobility,
coordination, and quality of life.

Eye Problems (Retinopathy): Elevated
blood sugar levels contribute to
diabetic retinopathy, a disorder that
damages blood vessels in the retina.
Untreated retinopathy can lead to
vision loss, blindness, and other eye
issues.

Kidney Damage (Nephropathy): Chronic hyperglycemia can damage the kidneys' blood vessels and impede their function, leading to diabetic nephropathy. This illness may develop into renal failure if not handled adequately.

Increased Infection Risk: High blood sugar impairs the immune system, making persons more susceptible to infections, particularly in the skin, urinary tract, and oral cavity. Poorly controlled diabetes can also impede wound healing and increase the risk of infections.

Slow Healing and Wound Complications: Chronic hyperglycemia can affect circulation and diminish the body's capacity to heal wounds, cuts, and ulcers. This raises the risk of infections, tissue damage, and consequences, especially in the lower extremities.

Complications During Pregnancy: High blood sugar levels during pregnancy (gestational diabetes) can lead to difficulties for both the mother and baby. These may include macrosomia (big birth weight), birth abnormalities, premature delivery, and a higher risk of

Type 2 diabetes later in life for the baby.

Mental Health Effects: Fluctuations in blood sugar levels and the stress of controlling diabetes can impair mental health. Individuals may experience mood fluctuations, anger, anxiety, depression, and cognitive deterioration over time.

High blood sugar levels pose major hazards and health implications, affecting multiple organ systems and raising the likelihood of long-term issues. Managing blood sugar efficiently through lifestyle adjustments, medication adherence, regular monitoring, and healthcare assistance is critical for decreasing these risks and improving overall health outcomes for those with diabetes or hyperglycemia.

Diabetes and Insulin Resistance

Diabetes is a chronic metabolic illness defined by increased blood sugar levels, either due to inadequate insulin synthesis, decreased insulin activity, or a combination of both. Insulin resistance is a major element in the development of Type 2 diabetes, where cells become less receptive to insulin's effects, leading to elevated blood sugar levels. In this section, we'll look into the relationship between diabetes and insulin resistance, investigating the mechanics, risk factors, and implications of this metabolic condition.

Understanding Insulin and Its Role: Insulin is a hormone generated by beta cells in the pancreas, necessary for glucose metabolism and blood sugar homeostasis. Its key functions include:

Facilitating Glucose Uptake: Insulin helps glucose enter cells, notably muscle, fat, and liver cells, where it is used for energy production and storage.

Suppressing Glucose manufacture: Insulin suppresses the liver's manufacture of glucose (gluconeogenesis) and increases glycogen synthesis, decreasing blood sugar levels.

Modulating Lipid and Protein Metabolism: Insulin regulates lipid storage (lipogenesis), protein synthesis, and cellular activities necessary for metabolism and cell function.

Insulin Resistance: Mechanisms and Causes:

a. Cellular Insensitivity: In insulin resistance, cells become less sensitive to insulin signals, particularly in muscle, liver, and adipose tissue. This inhibits glucose uptake and utilization, leading to high blood sugar levels.

b. Obesity and Inflammation: Excess body fat, especially visceral adipose tissue, contributes to inflammation, oxidative stress, and the release of cytokines that impair insulin signaling and induce insulin resistance.

c. Genetic Factors: Genetic predisposition can alter insulin sensitivity and contribute to the development of insulin resistance. Family history, ethnicity, and genetic differences in insulin-related genes play an impact.

Types of Diabetes Linked to Insulin Resistance:

a. Type 2 Diabetes: Insulin resistance is a hallmark of Type 2 diabetes, where cells fail to respond efficiently to insulin, leading to elevated blood sugar levels. Over time, beta cell malfunction may emerge, further limiting insulin production.

b. Gestational Diabetes: Pregnancy-related insulin resistance can lead to gestational diabetes, a transitory disease that increases the risk of problems for both the mother and baby.

Family History and Genetics: Genetic variables, family history of diabetes, and ethnic background increase susceptibility to insulin resistance and Type 2 diabetes.

Health Implications of Insulin Resistance and Diabetes:

a. High Blood Sugar (Hyperglycemia): Persistent hyperglycemia in diabetes can lead to long-term issues affecting the eyes, nerves, kidneys, and cardiovascular system.

b. Cardiovascular Disease: Insulin resistance and diabetes increase the risk of heart disease, stroke, hypertension, and atherosclerosis (hardening of arteries).

c. Nerve and Kidney Damage: Diabetic neuropathy (nerve damage) and nephropathy (kidney damage) are common effects of sustained high blood sugar levels and insulin resistance.

d. Eye Complications: Diabetic retinopathy, cataracts, and glaucoma are eye disorders related to diabetes and insulin resistance.

e. Metabolic Syndrome: Insulin resistance is a critical component of metabolic syndrome, a cluster of diseases including high blood pressure, excessive cholesterol levels, and abdominal obesity that raise cardiovascular risk.

Management and Prevention Strategies:

Lifestyle Modifications: Healthy nutrition, regular exercise, weight control, and smoking cessation can enhance insulin sensitivity and lower the risk of insulin resistance and diabetes.

Medication: Oral drugs (e.g., metformin, insulin sensitizers) and insulin therapy may be administered to regulate blood sugar levels and improve insulin function in diabetes.

Monitoring and Healthcare Support: Regular blood sugar monitoring, medical check-ups, and diabetes care regimens are crucial for those with insulin resistance or diabetes.

Insulin resistance is a crucial element in the development of Type 2 diabetes and is related to many metabolic problems and health hazards. Understanding the processes, risk factors, and health implications of insulin resistance and diabetes is critical for prevention, early detection, and effective management. Lifestyle adjustments, including healthy eating, physical activity, and weight control, have a crucial role in

improving insulin sensitivity,

regulating blood sugar levels, and

minimizing the risk of problems

associated with insulin resistance and

diabetes. Regular medical monitoring

and healthcare support are needed for

those at risk or diagnosed with insulin

resistance or diabetes to optimize their

health outcomes.

Long-Term Effects of Elevated Blood Sugar Levels

Elevated blood sugar levels, known as hyperglycemia, can have substantial long-term impacts on multiple organ systems and general health. Prolonged hyperglycemia, typically found in illnesses like diabetes, relates to a range of consequences that can dramatically influence the quality of life and health outcomes. In this section, we'll investigate the long-term implications of increased blood sugar levels and the potential issues linked with persistent hyperglycemia.

Diabetes Complications:

a. Cardiovascular Disease:

Atherosclerosis: Chronic hyperglycemia increases the production of fatty plaques in blood arteries, resulting in atherosclerosis. This increases the risk of heart attacks, strokes, and peripheral artery disease.

Hypertension: High blood sugar levels contribute to endothelial dysfunction and vascular inflammation, raising blood pressure and increasing

cardiovascular risk.

Cardiomyopathy: Prolonged

hyperglycemia can damage the heart

muscle, leading to cardiomyopathy and

heart failure.

b. Neuropathy: Peripheral Neuropathy:

Nerve damage induced by high blood

sugar levels can result in numbness,

tingling, discomfort, and weakness in

the extremities. This can affect

mobility, balance, and sensation.

Autonomic Neuropathy: Impaired nerve function can disturb involuntary physiological functions, impacting digestion, bladder control, heart rate, and blood pressure management.

c. Nephropathy: Diabetic Nephropathy: Chronic hyperglycemia destroys the kidneys' blood channels, leading to diabetic nephropathy. This can develop into renal failure, necessitating dialysis or transplantation.

Increased Proteinuria: Elevated blood sugar levels contribute to protein leakage in urine (proteinuria), a sign of kidney injury and compromised renal function.

d. Retinopathy: Diabetic Retinopathy: High blood sugar destroys blood vessels in the retina, leading to diabetic retinopathy. This can cause vision loss, blindness, and other eye issues if left untreated.

Macular Edema: Swelling of the macula (central region of the retina) due to fluid leaks from injured blood vessels, impairing central vision.

Metabolic Complications:

a. Obesity and Metabolic Syndrome:

Insulin Resistance: Prolonged hyperglycemia contributes to insulin resistance, a significant component in obesity and metabolic syndrome.

Abnormal Lipid Levels: High blood sugar levels can lead to dyslipidemia, characterized by raised triglycerides, reduced HDL cholesterol, and increased LDL cholesterol.

Abdominal Obesity: Excess visceral fat deposition, affected by insulin resistance, raises the risk of metabolic syndrome components like hypertension, dyslipidemia, and central obesity.

b. Oxidative Stress and Inflammation:
Cellular Damage: Chronic hyperglycemia enhances oxidative stress, leading to cellular damage, DNA mutations, and increased risk of chronic illnesses.

Inflammatory Response: Elevated blood sugar levels promote systemic inflammation, contributing to atherosclerosis, insulin resistance, and organ damage.

Mental Health and Cognitive
Implications:

a. Cognitive Decline: Prolonged
hyperglycemia is related to cognitive
impairment, memory decline, and a
higher risk of dementia and
Alzheimer's disease.

b. Mood Disorders: Fluctuations in
blood sugar levels can impair mood
stability, leading to anxiety, despair,
irritability, and psychological distress.

Delayed Healing and Wound
Complications:

Impaired Wound Healing: High blood sugar levels damage circulation, immunological function, and collagen synthesis, delaying wound healing and increasing the risk of infections, ulcers, and diabetic foot problems.

Pregnancy Complications:

Gestational Diabetes: Elevated blood sugar during pregnancy raises the risk of gestational diabetes, macrosomia (big birth weight), birth difficulties, and long-term health problems for the infant.

Maternal Health Risks: Uncontrolled hyperglycemia during pregnancy can lead to preeclampsia, cesarean birth, and a higher risk of Type 2 diabetes later in life for the mother.

The long-term implications of increased blood sugar levels, particularly in disorders like diabetes, cover a wide range of issues impacting cardiovascular health, nerve function, kidney function, vision, metabolism, mental health, wound healing, and pregnancy outcomes. Managing blood sugar correctly through lifestyle adjustments, medication adherence,

regular monitoring, and healthcare
assistance is critical for minimizing the
risk of long-term problems and
improving overall health outcomes for
those with diabetes or hyperglycemia.
Early detection, timely intervention,
and comprehensive treatment
techniques are critical for reducing the
impact of chronic hyperglycemia on
health and well-being.

CHAPTER 3

The Approach of the Glucose Revolution

The goal of the all-encompassing, scientifically supported Glucose Revolution method is to optimize blood sugar levels, support metabolic health, and prevent or treat diseases like metabolic syndrome, diabetes, and insulin resistance. To improve glucose regulation and general well-being, this approach highlights the significance of carbohydrate quality, glycemic index, lifestyle factors, and tailored nutrition. The main ideas and elements of the

Glucose Revolution diet and health philosophy will be discussed in this section.

Glycemic index and the quality of carbohydrates: a. What are carbohydrates? Carbohydrates are macronutrients that can be found in a variety of foods, such as grains, fruits, vegetables, legumes, and dairy products.

They supply energy in the form of calories and are essential for cellular processes, especially the metabolism of glucose.

a. The quality of carbohydrates: emphasize whole foods Place a focus on whole, unprocessed carbs like those found in whole grains, fruits, vegetables, and legumes that are high in fiber, minerals, vitamins, and phytochemicals.

Refined carbohydrates can cause blood sugar levels to jump and can lead to insulin resistance, so cut back on your intake of refined grains, sweets, and high-sugar processed meals.

c. Glycemic Index (GI): GI Ranking: Take into consideration a food's GI, or glycemic index, which indicates how quickly it raises blood sugar levels. To encourage consistent blood sugar control, select foods with a low to moderate GI.

Balanced Meals: To slow down digestion, lessen the impact of glycemic index, and increase satiety, combine carbohydrates with protein, healthy fats, and meals high in fiber.

Healthy Eating and Meal Planning: a. Macronutrient Balance: Protein Intake: To maintain muscular health, moderate blood sugar levels, and encourage

satiety, include lean proteins (such as
chicken, fish, lentils, and tofu) in
meals.

Healthy Fats: To support heart health,
insulin sensitivity, and nutrient
absorption, include unsaturated fats
(found in nuts, seeds, avocados, and
olive oil).

b. Foods High in Fiber: To slow down
digestion, enhance gut health, and
control blood sugar levels, choose
foods high in fiber, such as fruits,
vegetables, whole grains, and legumes.

Soluble Fiber: To help decrease cholesterol and enhance glycemic management, choose soluble fiber sources such as oats, beans, and flaxseeds.

c. Timing and Portion Control: Equilibrated Portions Control your portion sizes to prevent overindulging and preserve a healthy energy balance. Aim for well-balanced meals and snacks all day long.

Meal Timing: To avoid blood sugar spikes and sustain steady energy levels, take into account the timing and spacing of your meals. Frequent meal intervals can help with glucose management and metabolism.

Lifestyle and Physical Activity Factors:

a. Frequent Exercise: Cardiovascular Exercise Regular aerobic activity, such as jogging, cycling, or walking, can enhance insulin sensitivity, encourage muscle uptake of glucose, and support cardiovascular health.

Strength Training: To increase muscle development, speed up metabolism, and promote general fitness, incorporate strength training exercises (such as weightlifting and resistance training).

b. Stress Reduction Techniques: Stress Management Engage in stress-relieving practices to lower cortisol levels and promote emotional well-being, such as mindfulness, meditation, yoga, deep breathing, and relaxation techniques.

Sufficient Sleep: Make sure you get enough good sleep to support metabolic processes, balance hormones, and improve general health.

Observation and Tailored Strategy:

a. Blood Sugar Tracking: Frequent Assessment: Particularly for those with diabetes or insulin resistance, routinely check blood sugar levels to assess development, spot trends, and make necessary lifestyle or medication adjustments.

Continuous Glucose Monitoring (CGM): For up-to-date information on blood sugar patterns, the effects of meals, and individualized insights, take into account CGM devices.

b. Tailored Dietary Approach: Tailored Programs: Create individualized nutrition regimens based on each person's needs, preferences, health objectives, and medical problems by collaborating with healthcare professionals or nutritionists.

Dietary Advice: To maximize blood sugar control and general health, get advice on portion control, scheduling of meals, carb management, and dietary changes.

To optimize blood sugar levels, increase metabolic health, and improve overall well-being, the Glucose Revolution approach to health and nutrition places a strong emphasis on carbohydrate quality, glycemic index, balanced nutrition, physical exercise, stress management, and tailored treatment. People can enhance their quality of life, support glucose control, and avoid complications by using these lifestyle techniques and concepts. A proactive attitude to health management, consultation with nutritionists and healthcare professionals, and the successful use of the Glucose Revolution strategy are prerequisites for success.

Blood Sugar Balancing Principles

For general health, energy stability, and disease prevention—particularly when it comes to disorders like diabetes, insulin resistance, and metabolic syndrome—blood sugar regulation is essential. The mainstays of blood sugar regulation include lifestyle modifications, portion control, meal scheduling, and consistent monitoring. We'll go into the fundamentals of properly managing blood sugar in this part to promote metabolic health and well-being.

Select Light-Glycemic Foods:

Knowing the Glycemic Index (GI): The glycemic index calculates the pace at which food's carbs elevate blood sugar. Foods low in glycemic index (GI) gradually affect blood sugar levels, facilitating steady energy levels and insulin response.

Whole grains (such as oats, quinoa, and brown rice), legumes (like lentils, chickpeas, and beans), non-starchy vegetables, nuts, seeds, and fruits (including berries, apples, and citrus fruits) are a few examples of foods low in glycemic index (GI) content.

Make Fiber-Rich Foods a Priority:

The advantages of dietary fiber lower the absorption of glucose, slows down digestion, and increases feelings of fullness.

Sources of fiber: Include foods high in fiber in your meals and snacks, such as whole grains, legumes, nuts, seeds, vegetables, and fruits (even the ones with skin).

Mix Protein, Healthy Fats, and Carbohydrates:

Well-Balanced Meals: To improve satiety, slow down digestion, and stabilize blood sugar, pair carbohydrates with lean proteins (such as chicken, fish, tofu, and lentils) and healthy fats (such as avocado, olive oil, nuts, and seeds).

Examples of a well-balanced lunch might include quinoa paired with grilled chicken breast and roasted veggies tossed with olive oil.

Use Portion Control Techniques:

Properly Balanced Portions: To prevent overindulging and preserve energy balance, keep an eye on portion sizes. To help with portion control, use measurement devices or visual signals (such as a protein that is palm-sized or carbs that are fist-sized).

Steer clear of big meals: Large meals might cause blood sugar levels to rise quickly. Choose to eat smaller, more frequent meals or snacks all day long.

Restrict Added Sugars and Processed Meals: Take note of any added sugars in beverages, snacks, sauces, and processed meals. Select unprocessed, whole foods to cut down on sugar consumption and encourage stable blood sugar levels.

Examine the labels: Examine the sugar content of food labels and choose items with low or no added sugar.

Drink plenty of water and select low-calorie beverages:

Aqua: Stay hydrated and promote general health throughout the day by drinking lots of water. Drink less sugar-filled liquids, such as fruit juices, soda, and sweetened beverages.

Herbal Teas: For flavor without additional calories or sugar, sip herbal teas or infused water.

Incorporate Frequent Exercise:

Aerobic Exercise: To enhance insulin sensitivity, encourage muscle uptake of glucose, and maintain general metabolic health, regularly partake in aerobic exercises like walking, cycling, swimming, or dancing.

Strength Training: Use strength training activities to increase muscle growth, speed up metabolism, and regulate blood sugar.

Reduce Stress and Make Sleep a Priority:

Reducing Stress: Utilize stress-reduction methods to reduce cortisol levels and promote emotional well-being, such as mindfulness, meditation, deep breathing, yoga, or hobbies.

Aim for 7-9 hours of good sleep every night to enhance metabolic function, encourage restorative sleep, and manage hormones.

Track Your Blood Sugar Levels:

Frequent Observation: Patients with diabetes, insulin resistance, or factors that put them at risk should check their blood sugar levels as recommended by their healthcare experts.

Recognizing Patterns: To make educated dietary and lifestyle decisions, keep note of blood sugar trends, the effects of meals, and variables influencing glucose control.

Maintaining healthy blood sugar levels is essential for maintaining metabolic health and preventing disease. People can support stable blood sugar levels, improve insulin sensitivity, and enhance overall well-being by adhering to the principles of choosing low-glycemic foods, prioritizing fiber-rich meals, combining carbohydrates with protein and healthy fats, practicing portion control, limiting added sugars, staying hydrated, participating in regular physical activity, managing stress, prioritizing sleep, and monitoring blood sugar levels. For these principles to be successfully implemented and for ideal blood sugar balance to be achieved, healthcare professionals, nutrition experts, and proactive approaches to health management must be consulted.

Advantages of Keeping Blood Sugar Levels Stable

There are several advantages to maintaining steady blood sugar levels for general health, well-being, and illness avoidance. The following are the main benefits of maintaining blood sugar in a healthy range:

Increased Energy: The body and brain get a steady supply of energy from stable blood sugar levels. Preventing blood sugar spikes and crashes also helps avoid energy swings, which lessens feelings of exhaustion and sluggishness.

Improved Mental Clarity and Mood: Stable mood regulation and cognitive performance are supported by stable blood sugar levels. Preventing abrupt decreases in blood sugar, or hypoglycemia can help to improve mental clarity and attention by reducing mood swings, irritability, and brain fog.

Better Weight Management: Lower cravings for high-calorie or sugary foods and better appetite management are associated with stable blood sugar levels. This can lessen the chance of overeating and promote good eating habits, which can help with weight management attempts.

Lower Risk of Diabetes and Insulin Resistance: Type 2 diabetes and insulin resistance can both be avoided by keeping blood sugar levels steady. Stable blood sugar levels promote healthy insulin action and glucose metabolism, while persistently elevated blood sugar levels over time lead to insulin resistance.

Advantages for Heart Health: Because stable blood sugar levels lower the risk of atherosclerosis, hypertension, and heart disease, they improve cardiovascular health. Blood sugar fluctuations can cause stress on the cardiovascular system, whereas steady blood sugar levels promote heart health and vascular function.

Better Long-Term Metabolic Health: Maintaining stable blood sugar levels aids in the control of important metabolic functions such as hormone production, lipid metabolism, and cellular energy production. This can lower the risk of metabolic syndrome and have long-term advantages for metabolic health in general.

Improved Physical Performance: When engaging in physical exercise, stable blood sugar levels promote the best possible energy production. Blood sugar regulation has been shown to enhance endurance, stamina, and performance in athletes and active adults.

Improved Digestive Health: By encouraging regular bowel movements, lowering the risk of gastrointestinal pain, and preserving a healthy gut microbiota, stable blood sugar levels can improve digestive health.

Reduced Risk of Chronic Diseases: People who have stable blood sugar levels are less likely to develop long-term health issues like obesity, heart disease, some types of cancer, and neurological disorders. Effective blood sugar management promotes general well-being and lifespan.

Better Quality of Life: In general, having stable blood sugar levels lowers the chance of developing chronic illnesses, and increases energy, mental clarity, and physical health, all of which are factors in a higher quality of life. People might experience constant energy and vitality all day long because of it.

In summary, the advantages of keeping blood sugar steady go beyond short-term boosts to mood and energy levels to include long-term health outcomes, disease prevention, and general quality of life. People can maximize their blood sugar control and benefit from stable glucose metabolism by implementing healthy eating habits, engaging in regular physical activity, practicing stress management, and periodically monitoring their blood sugar levels.

CHAPTER 4

Nutritional Techniques for Blood Sugar Regulation

Blood sugar regulation is critical for general health, particularly for those with diabetes, insulin resistance, or those trying to avoid metabolic diseases. Dietary techniques are essential for properly controlling blood sugar. The following food tips are essential for maintaining blood sugar balance:

Select Light-Glycemic Foods:

Low-Glycemic Index (GI) items: Make sure your diet contains items low on the GI scale. These foods prevent blood sugar rises by releasing glucose into the system gradually. Whole grains (oats, quinoa, barley), legumes (lentils, chickpeas, kidney beans), non-starchy vegetables (broccoli, cauliflower, leafy greens), and the majority of fruits (strawberries, apples, citrus fruits) are a few examples.

Make Fiber-Rich Foods a Priority:

Soluble Fiber: To assist control blood sugar levels and slow down digestion, try to have enough soluble fiber in your diet. Oats, legumes, flaxseeds, chia seeds, vegetables like sweet potatoes and Brussels sprouts, and fruits like apples and pears are all excellent providers of soluble fiber.

Insoluble Fiber: To promote digestive health, include insoluble fiber from fruits, vegetables, and whole grains. Although it has no direct effect on blood sugar, insoluble fiber promotes satiety and a balanced metabolism.

Put Healthful Carbohydrates First:

Whole Grains: To take advantage of their higher fiber content and slower digestion, opt for whole grains rather than processed grains. Brown rice, quinoa, barley, whole wheat, and whole-grain pasta are a few examples.

Refined carbs should be consumed in moderation. This means consuming less sugar-filled drinks, white bread, pastries, sugary cereals, and other processed meals that include added sugars and refined grains. These may result in significant increases in blood sugar.

Add Lean Proteins:

Lean Protein Sources: Include low-fat dairy products, fish, chicken, tofu, tempeh, and legumes in your meals as lean protein sources. To minimize overeating and blood sugar swings, protein helps to normalize blood sugar levels and increases satiety.

Healthy Fats in Selected Amounts:

Consume monounsaturated and polyunsaturated fats in moderation, such as those found in avocados, nuts, seeds, olive oil, and fatty fish (sardines, salmon). Heart health, insulin sensitivity, and general metabolic balance are all supported by these lipids.

Limit Saturated and Trans Fats: Cut back on your consumption of processed meals, red meat, full-fat dairy products, and hydrogenated oils, which are present in fried foods. These fats may increase the risk of cardiovascular disease and insulin resistance.

Smart Portioning and Well-Balanced Meals:

Balanced Plate: Choose meals that are well-proportioned and feature a range of dietary groups. Arrange your plate such that non-starchy veggies make up half of it, lean protein makes up a quarter of it, and whole grains or healthy carbs make up the other quarter.

Snack Wisely: To avoid blood sugar increases in between meals, select nutritious snacks that include fiber, protein, and healthy fats. A tiny handful of nuts, hummus with vegetable sticks, and Greek yogurt with berries are a few examples.

Timing and Regularity of Meals:

Regular Meal Times: Try to eat at regular times each day to prevent blood sugar swings and overindulgence in later meals.

Eat mindfully by being aware of your hunger cues, taking your time, and ending when you're satisfied but not overstuffed. This can encourage improved blood sugar regulation and help avoid overindulging.

Drink Water to Remain Hydrated:

Hydration: To maintain proper metabolic function and stay hydrated,

sip lots of water throughout the day.
For sugar-free hydration, choose water,
herbal teas, or infused water instead of
sugar-filled beverages.

Check blood sugar and make necessary
adjustments:

Frequent Monitoring: As directed by
medical professionals, those with
diabetes or those who are monitoring
their blood sugar levels should check
their blood glucose levels regularly.
Make educated food decisions and any
necessary dietary adjustments using the
information provided.

Consult a Professional:

Speak with Registered Dietitians or Healthcare Providers: Seek advice from registered dietitians or healthcare providers if you have particular dietary requirements or medical issues with blood sugar regulation. They can help you achieve ideal blood sugar management, make customized food plans, and provide nutrition instruction.

You can maintain balanced blood sugar levels, enhance overall metabolic health, and lower the risk of issues related to blood sugar imbalances by implementing these dietary practices into your daily routine. Long-term achievement and maintenance of blood sugar balance depend on eating habits that are consistent, moderate, and thoughtful.

Choosing Foods Low in Glycemic Index (GI)

A measure of how quickly food's carbs elevate blood sugar is called the glycemic index (GI). Low-GI foods provide long-lasting energy and improve general health by gradually affecting blood sugar. By including low-GI items in your diet, you can promote long-term metabolic health, increase satiety, and stabilize blood sugar levels. Here are some guidelines and recommendations for selecting low-GI foods:

Knowing Your Glycemic Index:

Foods classified as low-GI are those with a GI value of 55 or lower. The sluggish digestion and absorption cause blood sugar levels to rise gradually.

Foods classified as moderate GI are those that have a GI rating of 56 to 69.

Their effect on blood sugar levels is mild.

Foods with a GI value of 70 or higher are classified as high-GI foods. They digest quickly, which quickly raises blood sugar levels.

Add Whole Grains:

Oats: Rich in soluble fiber, steel-cut, rolled, and oat bran are great low-GI alternatives that help to stabilize blood sugar levels by slowing down digestion.

Quinoa: This low-GI ancient grain provides a full complement of amino acids. It's a flexible ingredient that works well as a side dish or in salads and soups.

Brown Rice: Due to its increased fiber content and lower GI, brown rice is preferable to white rice. It is a wholesome mainstay in many international cuisines.

Make a Non-Starchy Vegetable Choice:

Leafy Greens: Low in calories and carbs, spinach, kale, Swiss chard, and other leafy greens are great options for preserving blood sugar balance.

Broccoli and cauliflower are low-GI, nutrient-dense cruciferous veggies. You can eat them grilled, steamed, or mixed into stir-fries.

Add Pulses and Legumes:

Lentils: Having a low GI, lentils are high in protein and fiber. They are used in soups, stews, and salads and can be used in place of meat in many different dishes.

Garbanzo beans sometimes referred to as chickpeas, are a rich source of fiber and plant-based protein because they have a low GI. They go well with roasted chickpeas, salads, curries, and hummus.

Include Lower-GI Fruits:

Berries: High in antioxidants, vitamins, and fiber, berries with a low GI include strawberries, blueberries, raspberries, and blackberries.

Pears and apples: These fruits are rich in soluble fiber and have a moderate GI, which helps control blood sugar levels and support digestive health.

Add in Lean Proteins and Fats:

Avocados: Avocados have a very low GI and are high in heart-healthy monounsaturated fats. They enhance the flavor and creaminess of salads, sandwiches, and dips.

Nuts and Seeds: Low in carbohydrates and having a low GI are almonds, walnuts, chia seeds, flaxseeds, and pumpkin seeds. They provide good lipids, fiber, and protein.

Pick Complete, Unprocessed Foods:

Whole Grain Bread and Pasta: For a lower GI and higher fiber content, choose whole grain or whole wheat bread and pasta over refined white options.

Steel-Cut Oats: Steel-cut oats have a lower GI than quick oats and make a filling, healthy breakfast choice.

Avert Processed and Sugary Foods:

Sugary Snacks and Drinks: Foods with a high GI that contain added sugars, like candy, pastries, sugary drinks, and desserts, can quickly raise blood sugar levels.

Processed Foods: Refined foods such as sugary cereals, white bread, white rice, and processed snacks typically have a higher GI. Whenever possible, go for whole, less processed options.

You can promote stable blood sugar levels, enhance general health, and lower your risk of metabolic illnesses by giving low-GI foods priority in your diet. Combine a range of whole grains, fruits, vegetables, legumes, healthy fats, and proteins to make wholesome, well-balanced meals that support optimal blood sugar regulation.

The proper ratios of carbs, proteins, and fats must be understood and incorporated into a diet to achieve a well-balanced diet. Every one of these macronutrients is essential for maintaining energy levels, metabolic processes, and general health. Here's how to successfully balance these macronutrients in your regular meals:

Glucose:

Goal: The body uses carbohydrates as its main energy source, particularly for the muscles and brain. Foods including cereals, fruits, vegetables, legumes, and dairy products contain them.

Carbohydrate Types:

Complex carbs can be found in whole grains, legumes, and vegetables. Because of their fiber content, which slows down digestion and stabilizes blood sugar levels, they offer lasting energy.

Simple carbs: Occurring in foods such as sugar, white bread, pastries, and sugary drinks, simple carbs should be consumed in moderation as they can quickly elevate blood sugar levels.

Keeping Carbs in Check:

For long-lasting energy and fiber, try to consume complex carbohydrates in most of your meals.

Select whole grains such as oats, brown rice, quinoa, and whole wheat bread that have undergone minimum processing.

Consume a range of vibrant fruits and vegetables to obtain vital antioxidants, vitamins, and minerals.

Proteins:

Proteins serve a variety of purposes, including the production of hormones and enzymes, immune system support, and tissue growth and repair. Meat, poultry, fish, eggs, dairy products, legumes, nuts, and seeds are among the foods that contain them.

Protein Types:

Fish, poultry, meat, eggs, and dairy products are examples of animal proteins. They supply every critical amino acid that the body requires.

Plant Proteins: Rich in fiber and antioxidants, plant proteins are typically lower in saturated fat and can be found in legumes (beans, lentils, chickpeas), tofu, tempeh, nuts, and seeds.

Proteins in Balance:

Every meal should contain a source of lean protein to support metabolic

health, muscle maintenance, and
satiety.

Choose lean meats, skinless chicken,
omega-3 fatty fish (sardines, mackerel,
and salmon), and plant-based proteins
(lentils and tofu).

Change up your protein sources every
week to guarantee a varied composition
of amino acids.

Lipids:

The purpose of dietary fats is to support
cell structure, hormone production,
energy storage, and the absorption of
nutrients, particularly fat-soluble

vitamins. Foods such as oils, butter, avocados, nuts, seeds, dairy products, and fatty fish contain them.

Different Fat Types:

Good Fats: You should give preference to monounsaturated and polyunsaturated fats in your diet because they are thought to be heart-healthy. They can be found in avocados, almonds, seeds, olive oil, and fatty fish (sardines, trout, and salmon).

Saturated Fats: To lower the risk of heart disease, consume saturated fats in moderation. They are present in animal products such as red meat, full-fat dairy, and some plant oils.

Trans Fats: Because they are bad for the heart, artificial trans fats, which are included in processed foods and partially hydrogenated oils, should be avoided.

Maintaining a Healthy Fat Balance:

Select your main sources of dietary fat from foods high in fat, such as nuts, seeds, avocado oil, olive oil, and fatty seafood.

Choose lean meats, cut visible fat, and use fat-free or low-fat dairy products to reduce your intake of saturated fats.

Examine food labels for trans fats and steer clear of those that use partially hydrogenated oils.

Proper Meals and Portion Sizes:

Make Balanced Plates: For the best nutrition and energy balance, try to incorporate all three macronutrients in each meal.

Portion management: To prevent overindulging and keep a healthy weight, practice portion management.

To properly portion out carbohydrates, proteins, and lipids, use visual clues or measurement equipment.

Meal Timing: To maintain steady energy levels and avoid blood sugar spikes and crashes, space meals and snacks out equally throughout the day.

Specific Needs:

Considerations: Age, sex, activity level, metabolic health, and medical disorders are a few examples of the variables that may affect an individual's nutritional needs.

Consultation: For individualized advice and meal planning, think about speaking with a registered dietitian or other healthcare professional if you have any health issues or special dietary needs.

You can promote general health, energy levels, and metabolic function by knowing the roles of fats, proteins, and carbs and ingesting them in balanced proportions. For a sustainable and healthful diet, emphasize complete, nutrient-dense foods, exercise portion control, and make well-informed decisions based on your unique needs and tastes.

Maintaining A Balance in Your Diet with Carbs, Proteins, And Fats

For general health and well-being, eating a balanced diet with sufficient amounts of fats, proteins, and carbs is essential. Every one of these macronutrients has a distinct purpose in the body, supporting different physiological processes, giving energy, and enhancing overall nutrition. You can successfully balance the amounts of fats, proteins, and carbs in your regular meals by doing the following:

The body uses carbohydrates as its main energy source, particularly for cognitive function and physical exercise. They fall into two primary categories:

Complex Carbohydrates: These can be found in fruits, vegetables, whole grains, and legumes. Their fiber content, which slows down digestion and aids in maintaining stable blood sugar levels, gives them lasting energy.

Simple carbs: Refined grains, processed snacks, and sugary meals are good sources of simple carbs. They can result in sharp rises in blood sugar levels due to their rapid digestion.

Keeping Carbs in Check:

Select whole grains (brown rice, quinoa, whole wheat), vegetables (broccoli, sweet potatoes, leafy greens), legumes (beans, lentils, chickpeas), and fruits (berries, apples, oranges) that are minimally processed.

Eat less simple carbs, such as those found in sugary cereals, candies, pastries, white bread, and sugary drinks.

If you want to increase satiety and control blood sugar, prioritize high-fiber foods.

Proteins: Building and mending tissues, bolstering immunological response, and generating hormones and enzymes all depend on proteins. They are made up of amino acids, some of which need to be supplied through diet as they are essential.

Sources of Animal Protein: Lean meats (turkey, chicken, lean beef, and pork cuts), fish, eggs, and dairy products (cottage cheese, Greek yogurt) are good sources of animal protein.

Plant Protein Sources: For plant-based protein sources, include legumes (beans, lentils, chickpeas), tofu, tempeh, nuts, seeds, and whole grains (quinoa, buckwheat).

Proteins in Balance:

Try to get some protein at every meal to help with satiety, metabolic support, and the health of your muscles.

Select lean meat slices, trim off any visible fat, and use baking, steaming, or grilling as your cooking techniques.

To guarantee a varied amino acid profile and optimize nutritional advantages, switch up your protein sources every week.

Fats: Dietary fats are necessary for hormone synthesis, nutrition absorption, energy storage, and cell structure. They are divided into two categories: good fats and less healthy fats.

Healthy Fat Sources: To obtain healthy fats, eat foods like avocados, nuts, seeds, olive oil, fatty fish (trout, mackerel, and salmon), and plant-based oils (walnut, flaxseed, and olive).

Fewer Healthful Fat Sources: Reduce your consumption of processed foods, full-fat dairy products, and red meat, which are high in saturated fats. Steer clear of the trans fats in margarine, baked products, and fried foods.

Maintaining a Healthy Fat Balance:

Give priority to heart health, brain function, and inflammation control in your diet by eating a diet high in healthy fats.

Because of their ability to reduce inflammation, incorporate sources of omega-3 fatty acids (found in fatty fish, flaxseeds, and chia seeds).

Saturated fats should be consumed in moderation, while trans fats should be avoided at all costs.

Proper Meals and Portion Sizes:

Make meals that are well-balanced and incorporate a range of items from the three major groups: fats, proteins, and carbohydrates.

To prevent overeating and preserve a healthy weight, practice portion management.

At every meal, include fruits and vegetables as a source of healthy fats, lean protein, and carbohydrates.

Aim for a plate that is half composed of veggies, 25% lean protein, and 25% whole grains or other healthful carbohydrates.

Customized Method:

When balancing macronutrients, take into account your personal nutritional needs, activity level, health objectives, and dietary preferences.

Speak with a qualified dietitian or other healthcare provider for individualized advice and meal planning that suits your needs and way of life.

You can achieve a balanced intake of carbs, proteins, and fats that supports optimal health, energy levels, and general well-being by adhering to these recommendations and making thoughtful dietary choices. For long-term health benefits, keep in mind to prioritize whole, nutrient-dense foods, exercise portion control, and maintain a varied and balanced diet.

The Function of Fiber in The Control of Blood Sugar

It is impossible to overestimate the importance of fiber in controlling blood sugar levels and how important it is to a balanced diet. It contributes significantly to the stabilization of blood sugar levels by slowing down the absorption of sugar into the bloodstream. This is an examination of the effects of fiber on the regulation of blood sugar:

Fiber Types:

In the digestive tract, soluble fiber turns into a gel-like material by dissolving in water. It can assist in blood sugar regulation and cholesterol reduction.

Insoluble Fiber: This type of fiber helps maintains regular bowel movements and digestive health by adding bulk to stool and refusing to dissolve in water.

Delaying Absorption and Digestion:

Because soluble fiber reduces the pace at which carbs are absorbed and digested, it is very advantageous for controlling blood sugar. Soluble fiber is found in foods high in fiber that gel in the digestive tract. Examples of these foods include oats, legumes, fruits like apples and oranges, and vegetables like carrots and Brussels sprouts. By delaying the stomach's emptying and sugar absorption, this gel causes blood sugar levels to rise gradually rather than suddenly.

While it has no direct effect on blood sugar, insoluble fiber supports regular bowel motions and general digestive health. This can help maintain a healthy gut environment, which can indirectly lead to improved blood sugar regulation.

An increase in insulin sensitivity

A diet high in fiber, particularly soluble fiber, has been demonstrated in studies to enhance insulin sensitivity. The hormone called insulin is in charge of transferring circulatory glucose into cells so that it can be utilized as an energy source. Blood sugar levels may rise as a result of cells developing insulin resistance. By enhancing insulin sensitivity, soluble fiber enables cells to absorb glucose more efficiently and sustain steady blood sugar levels.

Contentment and Control of Weight:

Foods high in fiber are frequently satisfying and can increase satiety, which lowers the risk of overindulging and consuming too many calories. Given that extra body weight can exacerbate insulin resistance and blood sugar abnormalities, this may help with weight management.

Suggested Consumption:

Adults should aim to consume at least 25-30 grams of total fiber daily, according to the American Heart Association. A varied diet rich in fruits, vegetables, whole grains, legumes, nuts, and seeds can help achieve this.

How to Include Fiber in Your Diet:

Brown rice, quinoa, whole wheat bread, and whole grain pasta are examples of whole grains that are preferable to refined grains.

Make sure your meals and snacks are full of fruits and veggies. Carrots, broccoli, spinach, oranges, bananas, berries, and apples are all great sources of fiber.

Add legumes to salads, soups, and main courses, such as beans, lentils, and chickpeas.

For an increase in fiber and nutrients, munch on nuts and seeds.

Aim for foods with a greater fiber content per serving and read food labels to identify products high in fiber.

Fiber and Hydration:

To avoid constipation and support good digestion, it's critical to drink enough water when consuming more fiber.

In conclusion, fiber slows down digestion, enhances insulin sensitivity, encourages fullness, and supports digestive health in general, all of which are critical for blood sugar regulation. Consuming a range of meals high in fiber will help you maintain improved blood sugar regulation and general health.

CHAPTER 5

Lifestyle Elements and Controlling Blood Sugar

Numerous lifestyle factors can either support stable blood sugar levels or exacerbate fluctuations and imbalances, which can have an impact on blood sugar management. Effective blood sugar management can be significantly aided by implementing healthy lifestyle practices. An outline of important lifestyle variables and how they affect blood sugar regulation is provided below:

Nutritional Decisions:

Balanced Meals: Eating meals that are well-proportioned with healthy fats, proteins, and carbs can help control blood sugar levels. Give priority to whole foods, including whole grains, fruits, vegetables, lean meats, and healthy fats.

Fiber-Rich Foods: Including foods high in fiber, such as fruits, vegetables, whole grains, legumes, nuts, and seeds, can help improve blood sugar regulation by slowing down the absorption of carbohydrates.

Reducing Sugary Items and Beverages: As sugary snacks, sweets, sodas, and other high-sugar items can quickly raise blood sugar levels, cut back on your intake of these.

Exercise:

Frequent Exercise: Taking regular walks, aerobic workouts, strength training, or other physical activities can help cells use glucose more efficiently and increase insulin sensitivity.

Consistency: To sustain long-term benefits for blood sugar management, strive for consistency in your workout regimen.

Controlling Weight:

Keeping a Healthy Weight: Excessive weight or obesity can increase blood sugar and insulin resistance. Blood sugar regulation benefits from weight management that combines regular exercise with a nutritious diet.

Losing Excess Weight: Even a small reduction in weight can help those who are overweight or obese by improving their blood sugar levels and general metabolic health.

Handling Stress:

Techniques for Reducing Stress: Take up stress-relieving exercises like yoga, tai chi, deep breathing, mindfulness meditation, or partaking in hobbies and enjoyable activities.

Good coping skills: Since long-term stress raises blood sugar levels, learn good coping skills to reduce stress.

Quality of Sleep:

Enough Sleep: Try to get seven to nine hours of good sleep each night.

Hormones that control hunger, glucose metabolism, and insulin sensitivity can be impacted by poor sleep hygiene and inadequate sleep.

Regular Sleep pattern: Even on weekends, keep a regular sleep pattern by going to bed and waking up at the same times every day.

Drinking plenty of water

Drink A Lot of Water: Maintaining stable blood sugar levels and supporting good renal function are two benefits of staying well-hydrated. Drink less sugary drinks and more water, herbal teas, or infused water.

Adherence to Medication:

Observe Doctor's Recommendations: If you have diabetes or another illness that necessitates taking medicine to control blood sugar, be sure you take your medications as directed by your doctor.

Monitor Blood Sugar Levels: As directed by your healthcare practitioner, periodically check your blood sugar levels to follow your progress and make any necessary modifications.

Drinking of Alcohol:

Moderation: If you drink alcohol, make sure you know how it affects your blood sugar levels and only drink in moderation. Blood sugar swings can be brought on by alcohol, so it's critical to keep an eye on your consumption and make wise decisions.

Frequent Medical Examinations:

Regular Check-ups: Make an appointment for routine health check-ups with your physician to monitor your blood sugar levels, evaluate your general health, and modify your treatment plan or lifestyle as needed.

You can improve blood sugar control and general health by adopting these lifestyle variables into your regular activities. Maintaining stable blood sugar levels and lowering the risk of consequences from blood sugar imbalances need consistency, moderation, and making good decisions.

The Value of Engaging in Exercise

Maintaining general health and well-being requires continuing physical activity. It includes any type of activity that uses up energy and works your muscles, such as walking, gardening, and structured exercise regimens like swimming, jogging, or strength training. Physical activity has many advantages for both physical and mental health, therefore its significance goes far beyond merely physical fitness. The following are some main justifications for why exercise is vital:

Enhances Cardiovascular Health: Regular exercise strengthens the heart and enhances cardiovascular health. It promotes better circulation, lowers blood pressure, and lowers the risk of heart disease, all of which contribute to a healthy cardiovascular system in general.

Improves Muscle Strength and Flexibility: Exercise, especially resistance training, helps to increase muscle strength and endurance. Additionally, it increases joint mobility, flexibility, and total functional capacity, which facilitates the performance of daily duties.

Supports Weight Management: By boosting metabolism, burning calories, and encouraging the maintenance of lean muscle mass, regular physical exercise is essential for weight management. It can enhance body composition, support attempts to lose weight and stop weight gain.

Enhances Metabolic Health: Exercise lowers the risk of metabolic diseases like type 2 diabetes, increases insulin sensitivity, and helps control blood sugar levels. By decreasing triglycerides and increasing "good" HDL cholesterol, it also helps to improve lipid profiles.

Strengthens Bones and Joints: Activities involving weight bearing, such as dancing, jogging, walking, and strength training, assist in increasing bone density, strengthen bones, and lower the risk of osteoporosis. Because it lowers the risk of arthritis and promotes cartilage health, physical activity also helps to maintain joint health.

Improves Mental Well-Being: Engaging in physical activity has a positive impact on one's mental and emotional health. It helps lessen the symptoms of sadness and anxiety, releases feel-good hormones called endorphins to elevate mood, enhances brain clarity and general cognitive function, and improves the quality of sleep.

Enhances Longevity and Quality of Life: Several research studies have demonstrated the link between regular physical exercise and a longer lifetime, as well as a lower chance of chronic illnesses and early death. By enhancing physical function, independence, and general vitality, it raises the quality of life.

Lessens Stress and Increases Resilience: Exercise is a natural way to reduce stress. It increases resilience to everyday stressors, encourages relaxation, and lowers levels of stress chemicals like cortisol.

Enhances Immune System: Studies have indicated that moderate-intensity exercise increases immunity and lowers the risk of infections and chronic illnesses. It promotes the general health of the immune system, lowers inflammation, and improves immunological surveillance.

Social Engagement and Connection: Opportunities for social interaction, companionship, and a sense of belonging are offered by a variety of physical activities, including team sports, group exercise classes, and outdoor pursuits. These aspects of physical activity are crucial for one's mental and emotional health.

One of the best decisions you can make for your health is to include regular physical activity in your lifestyle. Getting moving every day, participating in organized workouts, or engaging in enjoyable hobbies can all contribute to a more active lifestyle, which can improve your mental and physical health along with your overall standard of living.

Techniques for Stress Management

In the fast-paced world of today, stress management is becoming more and more crucial to preserving general health and quality of life. Prolonged stress can negatively affect one's physical and emotional well-being, resulting in a variety of health problems such as anxiety, depression, hypertension, and compromised immune systems. Fortunately, you may increase your resilience and learn how to handle stress by using one of the many useful stress management techniques. Consider the following strategies:

Breathing Techniques:

Diaphragmatic breathing, sometimes referred to as belly breathing, is a method that entails taking deep, slow breaths, filling your lungs, and stretching your diaphragm. For four counts, take a deep breath through your nose, hold it, and then gently release the breath through your mouth for four counts.

Box breathing involves taking a deep breath, holding it for four counts, exhaling for four counts, pausing for four counts, and then starting the cycle over. This regular breathing technique can ease nervous system tension and lower stress levels.

Progressive Muscle Relaxation (PMR): To encourage relaxation and lessen the tenseness of your muscles brought on by stress, PMR entails tensing and relaxing various muscle groups in your body. Begin by tensing a particular muscle group (for example, your shoulders or fists) for a brief period, then let go and fully relax. Work your way from head to toe through each muscle group.

Meditation with mindfulness:

Focused Attention Meditation: Set your attention on a single point, such as your breath, a mantra, or a particular sense, like the sensation of your feet touching the floor. Gently and without passing judgment, return your attention to the main issue when you become sidetracked.

Body Scan Meditation: Shut your eyes and carefully examine your entire body, noticing any points of stress or discomfort. Breathe into these sensations as you become aware of them, and with each exhale, deliberately release tension.

Tai Chi and Yoga:

Yoga: Yoga is a powerful stress-relieving practice that integrates physical movement, breath awareness, and mindfulness. Asana (corpse position), downward-facing dog, and child's pose are among the poses that help ease tension and encourage calm.

Tai Chi: Mindfulness, deep breathing, and fluid, leisurely motions are the main components of this peaceful martial art. Tai chi helps lessen stress and anxiety while enhancing balance, flexibility, and mental clarity.

Frequent Exercise: Physical activity regularly, such as walking, jogging, cycling, dancing, or playing sports, can help lower stress levels and elevate mood. The body's inherent feel-good hormones, endorphins, are released when you exercise and can improve your general mood.

Choosing a Healthier Lifestyle:

Dietary Balance: Consume a diet high in fruits, vegetables, whole grains, lean meats, and healthy fats. Steer clear of excessive amounts of alcohol, sugar, and caffeine as they can aggravate anxiety and tension.

Sufficient Sleep: Make it a priority to obtain seven to nine hours of good sleep every night to promote both mental and physical recuperation, lessen exhaustion, and increase stress tolerance.

Time management: To lessen emotions of stress and overwhelm, prioritize your work, delegate where you can, and manage your time well.

Social Support and Connection: Keep up close ties with your loved ones, and friends, and support people. Stress can be reduced and emotional support can be obtained by talking about your feelings, asking for guidance or an alternative viewpoint, and sharing experiences.

Activities that Encourage Mindfulness and Relaxation: Take part in activities that encourage mindfulness and relaxation, such as doing crafts or art, writing, going on nature walks, or listening to soothing music.

Seeking Professional Support: You should think about getting help from a therapist, counselor, or mental health professional if your stress becomes unbearable or chronic. They can offer you direction, coping mechanisms, and therapeutic interventions to assist with stress management.

Self-Care Routines: Give your mind, body, and soul the nourishment they need. This could be establishing boundaries, saying no when it's necessary, taking pauses, practicing self-compassion, taking pleasure in relaxing activities, and setting boundaries.

You may strengthen your coping mechanisms, increase your resilience, and lessen the detrimental effects of stress on your general health and well-being by implementing these stress management practices into your daily routine. Try out various tactics to see which one suits you the best, and keep in mind that self-care and regular practice are essential elements of successful stress management.

The Effects of Good Sleep On Blood Sugar

In addition to being crucial for maintaining general health and well-being, getting enough sleep is also important for controlling blood sugar levels and other physiological processes. The complicated relationship between blood sugar and sleep is that insulin sensitivity and glucose metabolism are adversely affected by inadequate or poor-quality sleep. This study examines the relationship between good sleep and blood sugar regulation:

Hormone Regulation: Getting enough sleep is essential for preserving the proper ratio of the hormones insulin and cortisol, which are key players in controlling blood sugar.

Insulin: Lack of sleep or inadequate sleep quality can cause insulin resistance, a condition in which cells lose their sensitivity to insulin signals, raising blood sugar levels.

Cortisol: Sleep deprivation can affect cortisol levels, which are a stress hormone that can lead to raised blood sugar and insulin resistance when it is elevated over time.

Effect on the Metabolism of Glucose:

Utilization of Glucose: The body repairs and regenerates its cells when you sleep, and this includes the utilization of glucose. Good sleep facilitates proper glucose metabolism, which guarantees that cells efficiently absorb glucose for energy.

Sleep has an impact on liver function, which in turn helps to keep blood sugar levels steady. Getting enough sleep helps the body store and release glycogen in the right amounts, which keeps the liver from producing too much glucose.

Sensitivity to Insulin:

Improved Sensitivity: Getting enough sleep improves insulin sensitivity, which makes it possible for cells to react to insulin's effects more efficiently and encourages the best possible blood sugar regulation.

Diminished Insulin Resistance: On the other hand, insufficient sleep or irregular sleep schedules can cause insulin resistance, which makes it difficult for cells to use glucose effectively and eventually raises blood sugar levels.

Control of Appetite:

Hormones that Control Appetite: Hormones like ghrelin and leptin are influenced by sleep. These hormones can be upset by sleep deprivation, which can raise hunger, cause cravings for high-calorie foods, and perhaps lead to overeating, which can raise blood sugar levels.

Late-Night Eating: Since late meals can alter insulin sensitivity and glucose metabolism, irregular sleep patterns or late-night eating might further impair blood sugar management.

Stress and Inflammation:

Inflammatory Response: Systemic inflammation is linked to insulin resistance and decreased glucose metabolism. It can be caused by inadequate or poor sleep.

Stress Response: Lack of sleep can also set off a stress response that raises cortisol levels and messes with insulin sensitivity and blood sugar balance.

Ideas to Enhance the Quality of Your Sleep:

Create a Regular Sleep Schedule: To keep your body's internal clock in check, go to bed and wake up at the same time every day, including on the weekends.

Establish a Calm Bedtime Routine: To help your body and mind get ready for sleep, engage in relaxing activities like deep breathing, meditation, light yoga, or reading a book before bed.

Optimize Your Sleep Environment: Set up a cool, dark, and peaceful sleeping space with a cozy mattress and pillows.

Limit Screen Time: Try to avoid using screens (such as phones, tablets, laptops, and TVs) right before bed because blue light can interfere with the generation of melatonin and cause sleep disturbances.

Steer Clear of Stimulants: Restrict your intake of caffeine and nicotine, especially in the hours before bed, as these chemicals may disrupt your sleep.

Handle Stress: To lower stress levels and encourage better sleep, use stress-reduction strategies including mindfulness, and relaxation techniques, or consult a therapist or counselor.

You can enhance insulin sensitivity, promote overall metabolic health, and have a positive effect on blood sugar regulation by making quality sleep a priority and developing appropriate sleep habits. A healthy lifestyle is mostly dependent on getting regular, restful sleep, which is also essential for maintaining ideal blood sugar control and general well-being.

CHAPTER 6

Keeping an eye on and recording blood sugar levels

It is imperative for those with diabetes, prediabetes, or those at risk of developing these disorders to track and monitor their blood sugar levels. Frequent monitoring enables efficient management and the avoidance of issues by assisting patients and medical professionals in understanding how the body reacts to certain stimuli, including food, exercise, drugs, and lifestyle choices. An outline of the significance of blood sugar monitoring and practical methods for doing so is provided below:

The Value of Observation

Optimal Blood Sugar Control: By keeping an eye on blood sugar levels, people may evaluate how well their blood sugar is controlled right now and take well-informed actions to keep it there.

Medication Adjustments: Regular monitoring helps assess the efficacy of treatment and permits necessary modifications for people taking insulin or oral hypoglycemic medicines.

Preventing Complications: Regular blood sugar monitoring can help identify patterns or fluctuations in blood sugar levels early on, which lowers the risk of hyperglycemia (high blood sugar) and hypoglycemia (low blood sugar), as well as potential consequences like kidney disease, cardiovascular problems, and nerve damage.

Lifestyle Management: Monitoring blood sugar levels helps people take proactive steps to improve their management by giving them important information about how their food, exercise, stress levels, sleep patterns, and other lifestyle factors affect blood sugar control.

Techniques for Surveillance:

Blood glucose meters: These handheld gadgets use a tiny drop of blood drawn with a finger stick to measure blood sugar levels. They are frequently used for everyday home monitoring and offer fast results.

Continuous Glucose Monitoring (CGM) Systems: CGM systems assess blood glucose levels constantly day and night using sensors inserted beneath the skin. They offer data, trends, and warnings for high and low blood sugar levels in real-time.

Blood sugar averages for the preceding two to three months are determined by the A1C test. It is usually carried out every three to six months and offers a snapshot of long-term blood sugar control.

Urine testing: Although less frequent than blood testing, urine tests can be used to assess blood sugar levels; nevertheless, the results are not as precise or instantaneous as those obtained by blood glucose monitoring techniques.

Monitoring Frequency:

Type of Diabetes: Individual treatment regimens and the type of diabetes (Type 1, Type 2, gestational diabetes) may have an impact on how frequently an individual is monitored.

Individual Needs: Medical professionals frequently suggest customized monitoring plans based on the needs of each patient. These plans may include daily, pre- or post-meal, overnight, or continuous monitoring using continuous glucose monitoring (CGM) devices.

Monitoring Techniques:

Blood Sugar Log: Record blood sugar readings together with information on the time of day, meals, medications, physical activity, symptoms, and any other factors that can affect blood sugar levels in a blood sugar log or via a mobile app.

Pattern Recognition: Examine blood sugar data over an extended period to spot trends, patterns, and variables that influence blood sugar regulation. Keep an eye out for regular highs and lows, eating or activity routines, and any changes that should be made to prescription drugs or lifestyle choices.

Communication with Healthcare Team: During routine check-ins or appointments, share blood sugar data and monitoring logs with your healthcare team. Work together to reach well-informed decisions on blood sugar management targets, lifestyle modifications, and treatment modifications.

Some Advice for Skillful Observation:

Regularly check your blood sugar levels as directed by your healthcare professional, whether that's once a week, every day, or as frequently as needed.

Accuracy: To guarantee accurate findings, use dependable CGM systems or blood glucose meters and adhere to recommended testing procedures.

Education: Acquire the skills necessary to evaluate blood sugar readings, comprehend goal ranges, spot hypo- or hyperglycemia symptoms, and know when to call for help.

Documentation: To monitor progress and make wise decisions, keep thorough records of blood sugar readings, prescription drugs, meals, physical activity, symptoms, and other pertinent data.

Making Use of Technology

Mobile Apps: There are a plethora of apps available for tracking blood sugar levels, trend analysis, prescription and test reminders, and sharing data with healthcare providers.

Smart Devices: Data from certain blood glucose meters and CGM systems can be wirelessly synced to computers, tablets, and smartphones, making it simpler to monitor and control blood sugar levels while on the go.

Awareness and Empowerment:

Individuals who regularly check and monitor their blood sugar levels are better able to control their diabetes, become more self-aware, and make decisions that will enhance their health. To consistently improve blood sugar control and general well-being, it's critical to stay up to date on new monitoring tools, methods, and policies.

People with diabetes or prediabetes can live healthier lives by managing their blood sugar levels more effectively, lowering their risk of problems, and making greater use of available technology. These strategies include regular monitoring, precise tracking techniques, efficient communication with healthcare providers, and leveraging accessible technology.

Self-Observation Methods

Self-monitoring strategies are useful
tools for those who want to keep tabs
on different facets of their behavior,
health, or progress toward particular
objectives. These methods entail
keeping track of pertinent information
about one's physical, mental, or
emotional health through observation
and recording. An examination of self-
monitoring methods and their
advantages is provided below:

Monitoring Fitness and Health:

Physical Activity: Record the kind,
length, and intensity of your daily or

weekly workouts, as well as any accomplishments you may have made. When working out, track your steps, distance traveled, calories burned, and heart rate using fitness apps or wearable technology.

Nutrition and Diet: Keep a food journal to track your intake of macronutrients (carbs, proteins, and fats), meals, snacks, and portion sizes. Keep a watch on your calorie intake, hydration levels, and any dietary trends or triggers that may have an impact on your health.

Sleep Patterns: Monitor the length, quality, and timing of your slumber as well as any variables that may affect it (e.g., caffeine intake, screen time before bed). To keep track of sleep patterns, disruptions, and stages over time, use sleep-tracking devices or applications.

Stress and Mood: Keep an eye on your stress levels, mood swings, emotional triggers, coping mechanisms, and relaxing or well-being-promoting activities. To document thoughts, feelings, and actions linked to mental and emotional well-being, keep a journal or use applications that measure mood.

Vital indicators and health parameters:

Blood Pressure: If you have hypertension or are at risk of high blood pressure, use a home blood pressure monitor to frequently measure your results.

Blood Sugar Levels: Self-monitoring blood sugar levels with a glucometer or continuous glucose monitoring (CGM) device is crucial for controlling blood sugar in people with diabetes or prediabetes.

Weight and Body Composition: To track your progress toward weight management or fitness goals, keep track of changes in your body weight, measures, body fat percentage, and muscle mass.

Tracking Behavior and Habits:

Quitting smoking: Monitor your smoking behaviors, desires, triggers, and progress toward your goals if you're attempting to cut back on tobacco usage or quit smoking.

Medication Adherence: Track medication dosages, regimens, adverse effects, and compliance with recommended therapies by keeping a medication journal. To keep organized, use apps for medication management or set reminders.

Hydration: Keep an eye on your regular intake of fluids, water consumption, and level of hydration to make sure you're getting enough water, especially during hot weather or strenuous exercise.

Setting Objectives and Monitoring
Results:

SMART Goals: Establish SMART
(specific, measurable, attainable,
relevant, and time-bound) objectives
for your diet, exercise, stress relief, and
other areas of interest.

Progress tracking: Using graphs, charts,
or other visual aids to track trends,
milestones, failures, and
accomplishments, evaluate and update
your goals' progress regularly. Reward
accomplishments and make necessary
strategy adjustments to keep on course.

Apps and Technology:

Mobile Apps: To simplify self-monitoring, obtain individualized insights, receive reminders, and sync data across devices, make use of wellness trackers, habit-building apps, mood journals, health and fitness apps, and other digital tools.

Wearable Technology: To assist self-monitoring efforts, think about utilizing wearable technology, such as fitness trackers, smartwatches, or health monitors that provide real-time data tracking, activity reminders, heart rate monitoring, sleep analysis, and other functions.

The advantages of self-monitoring

Self-monitoring encourages self-awareness, mindfulness, and accountability for actions, decisions, and results connected to one's health.

Patterns and Triggers: Monitoring data over an extended period facilitates the identification of trends, patterns, correlations, and possible triggers that affect behavior, habits, and general well-being.

Goal Achievement: People can work toward attaining desired results, making positive changes, and

maintaining healthy behaviors over the long term by setting goals, keeping track of their progress, and making data-informed decisions.

Communication with Healthcare Professionals: During consultations, self-monitored data can be shared with healthcare professionals to help with discussions, evaluate progress, modify treatment plans, and get individualized advice or recommendations.

Using self-monitoring strategies can be a helpful tactic for encouraging self-care, making wise decisions, and reaching your health and wellness objectives, regardless of your goals—improving mental health, managing chronic conditions, fostering healthier habits, or becoming fitter. Customize your self-monitoring strategy to your requirements, interests, and preferences. Make use of resources and technology to assist you on your path toward self-care.

Managing Blood Sugar Using Technology

The way people control their blood sugar levels has been completely transformed by technological advancements, particularly for those who have diabetes or prediabetes. There are numerous technical instruments and gadgets available to efficiently track, monitor, analyze, and manage blood sugar. Here is an examination of the advantages of using technology for blood sugar control:

Blood Pressure Monitors:

Conventional Meters: Blood glucose meters (BGMs) are handheld instruments that use a finger stick to draw a tiny drop of blood to test blood sugar levels. They enable people to check their blood sugar levels at home or while they're on the go because they produce findings right away.

Advanced Features: Current BGMs have programmable settings for alarms and reminders, memory storage for previous readings, average glucose calculations, and data communication to computers or cell phones for trend tracking.

Systems for Continuous Glucose Monitoring (CGM):

Continuous Monitoring: CGM devices monitor blood glucose levels constantly day and night using sensors inserted beneath the skin. They offer data, trends, and warnings for high and low blood sugar levels in real-time.

Data Visualization: CGM systems provide capabilities for data visualization, such as reports, glucose trends, and patterns, which can be seen on tablets, smartphones, or special receiver devices. This supports people's and healthcare professionals' data-driven decision-making around blood sugar control.

Insulin Pumps:

combined devices: A closed-loop system that automatically modifies insulin delivery depending on real-time glucose measurements is created when certain insulin pumps are combined with CGM devices. This technique helps improve blood sugar regulation and lower the risk of hypo- or hyperglycemia. It is also referred to as automated insulin delivery or hybrid closed-loop technology.

Intelligent Insulin Pumps: State-of-the-art insulin pumps may be equipped with intelligent features including mobile app connectivity, bolus calculators, configurable settings, and predictive algorithms for remote monitoring and administration.

Digital platforms and mobile applications:

Health applications: There are a plethora of health applications available with features tailored exclusively for

managing blood sugar, including tools
for data analysis, glucose tracking,
meal recording, medication reminders,
and activity tracking.

Remote Monitoring: Through the use
of certain apps and platforms, people
can share their blood sugar readings
with family members, caregivers, or
medical professionals for cooperative
support and management.

Educational materials: People can learn
more about managing their diabetes,
making lifestyle adjustments, and
following best practices by visiting

digital platforms, which frequently include advice, articles, community forums, and educational materials.

Virtual Care and Telemedicine:

Remote Consultations: For individualized advice, treatment modifications, and support, people can use telemedicine platforms to schedule virtual consultations with healthcare professionals such as endocrinologists, diabetic educators, dietitians, and pharmacists.

Programs for Remote Monitoring: Several healthcare providers allow patients to participate in virtual coaching or self-management initiatives, upload blood sugar readings regularly, and receive feedback.

Analyses of Data and Conclusions:

Data analytics: Sophisticated algorithms and software examine blood sugar data to spot abnormalities, trends, and patterns. They then offer recommendations and actionable insights for improving blood sugar control.

Predictive Modeling: By using data from the present to predict blood sugar levels in the future, certain technological platforms enable people with diabetes to take proactive care of their condition and avoid swings.

Advantages of Technology Use:

Increased Accuracy: Thanks to advancements in technology, blood sugar monitoring is now more dependable and accurate, with fewer mistakes and more exact measurements.

Real-Time Monitoring: In the event of hypo- or hyperglycemia, CGM devices and smartphone apps offer real-time

monitoring, warnings, and notifications
for prompt actions.

Data Tracking and Trends: People and
healthcare professionals can discover
patterns, make data-driven decisions,
and modify treatment plans as
necessary thanks to technology's
continuous data tracking, trend
analysis, and visualization capabilities.

Enhanced Self-Management: By using
technology, people can better control
their blood sugar levels by making
educated decisions, setting objectives,
monitoring their progress, and

increasing their adherence to treatment plans.

Remote Support and Collaboration: By facilitating communication, education, and the overall management of diabetes, telemedicine, digital platforms, and remote monitoring promote collaboration among patients, healthcare professionals, and support networks.

Many advantages come with integrating technology into blood sugar management, such as increased self-management skills, real-time monitoring, data analysis, and accuracy. Through the use of cutting-edge technological tools and resources, people with diabetes can lower their risk of complications, improve their blood sugar regulation, and enjoy healthier, more independent lives.

CHAPTER 7

Blood Sugar Balance Recipes

The following recipes aim to support blood sugar regulation and general well-being:

Quinoa and Veggie Stir-Fry: Add the following ingredients: 1 cup of washed quinoa

two cups of veggie broth or water

One tablespoon of olive oil

one sliced onion

two minced cloves of garlic

One chopped bell pepper

One sliced zucchini

one cup florets of broccoli

One carrot, thinly sliced

Two teaspoons of tamari or low-sodium soy sauce

One-teaspoon rice vinegar

one tsp finely chopped ginger

To taste, add salt and pepper.

To garnish, use fresh cilantro.

Guidelines:

Quinoa should be combined with broth or water in a medium saucepan. After bringing it to a boil, lower the heat, cover, and simmer the quinoa for 15 to 20 minutes, or until it is tender and the liquid has been absorbed.

Over medium heat, warm the olive oil in a large skillet. Add the garlic and onion, and cook until aromatic.

To the skillet, add the bell pepper, carrot, broccoli, and zucchini. Cook the vegetables in a stir-fry until they become soft and crispy.

Combine the soy sauce, rice vinegar, grated ginger, salt, and pepper in a small bowl. After adding the sauce to the veggies, mix everything.

After the quinoa has cooked, add it to the skillet and mix everything until thoroughly combined and hot.

Before serving, garnish with fresh cilantro.

Salmon Baked with Asparagus:

Ingredients: 4 fillets of salmon

One cut bunch of asparagus

Two tsp olive oil

One sliced lemon

two minced cloves of garlic

One tsp of dried dill to taste, add salt
and pepper.

 Guidelines:

Turn the oven on to 400°F, or 200°C.
For lining a baking sheet, use
parchment paper.

Arrange the asparagus around the
salmon fillets once they are placed on
the baking pan.

Pour some olive oil over the asparagus
and fish. Add salt, pepper, dried dill,
and minced garlic for seasoning.

Top each salmon fillet with a slice of
lemon.

Bake the salmon for 15 to 20 minutes
in a preheated oven, or until it is
cooked through and flake easily with a
fork.

If preferred, top the hot dish with extra
lemon wedges.

Salad with chickpeas and spinach:

Components:

One can of washed and drained
chickpeas

Two cups of raw spinach

one chopped cucumber

One chopped tomato

1/4 of a red onion, cut thinly

1/4 cup of feta cheese, crumbled (optional)

Two tsp olive oil

One-third cup of balsamic vinegar

One tsp honey or maple syrup

To taste, add salt and pepper.

Guidelines:

Chickpeas, spinach, cucumber, tomato, red onion, and feta cheese should all be combined in a big bowl.

To create the dressing, combine the olive oil, balsamic vinegar, honey (or

maple syrup), salt, and pepper in a small bowl.

After pouring the dressing over the salad, toss to ensure an even coating.

Serve right away as a nutrient-dense, refreshing salad.

Rich in fiber, lean protein, good fats, and complex carbohydrates, these dishes support optimal blood sugar regulation and general well-being.

Savor these tasty and nourishing dishes
as part of a balanced diet that aims to
support optimum health.

Ideas for Healthful Meals

Skewers of grilled chicken and
vegetables:

Components:

Cubes of skinless, boneless chicken
breasts

Red, yellow, and green bell peppers,
chopped into bits

sliced red onion into wedges

rosy tomatoes

Sliced zucchini

Olive oil

Juice from lemons

Powdered garlic

Add pepper and salt.

Water-soaked wooden skewers

Guidelines:

Grill at a medium-high temperature.

Vegetables and poultry pieces are alternately threaded onto skewers.

To make a marinade, combine the olive oil, lemon juice, garlic powder, salt, and pepper in a small bowl.

Apply the marinade on the skewers. Cook the kebabs for ten to twelve minutes, rotating them halfway

through, or until the chicken is thoroughly cooked and the veggies are soft.

Warm up and serve with brown rice or quinoa on the side.

Buddha Bowl for Vegetarians:

Ingredients:

Brown rice or cooked quinoa

Cubed and roasted sweet potatoes

Broccoli florets steam-cooked

Garlic-sautéed spinach

Roasted chickpeas with spices

slices of avocado

Dressing with tahini or hummus

Fresh herbs for garnish, such as parsley

and cilantro

Directions: Place cooked brown rice or

quinoa in a bowl to serve as the

foundation.

On top, arrange portions of roasted sweet potatoes, steaming broccoli, sautéed spinach, roasted chickpeas, and avocado slices.

Pour over some tahini dressing or hummus.

Before serving, add a fresh herb garnish.

Ingredients for Salmon and Quinoa Salad: baked or grilled salmon fillets cooked quinoa

Mixed greens: kale, spinach, and arugula

Halves of cherry tomatoes, sliced cucumbers

Red onion, finely sliced avocado, diced goat or Feta cheese (if desired)

Dressing with lemon vinaigrette

Guidelines:

Make the fish grilled or baked, depending on your tastes.

Cooked quinoa, mixed greens, cucumber, red onion, avocado, and cheese (if using) should all be combined in a big bowl.

Toss to ensure even coating after adding a drizzle of lemon vinaigrette dressing.

Add grilled salmon fillets to the salad.

Serve as a filling and healthy meal.

Chicken wrap with a Mediterranean flair:

Components:

Chicken breasts that are grilled or shred

Spinach or whole-wheat tortilla wraps

Dipsticks Tzatziki

cucumber slices

Half a cherry tomato

Slices of red onion, thinly

Fresh arugula or spinach leaves

Guidelines:

Top a tortilla wrap with tzatziki sauce
and hummus.

Arrange the following in layers: grilled
chicken, cherry tomatoes, red onion,
cucumber slices, and fresh spinach or
arugula leaves.

After tightly rolling the wrap, cut it in half.

Accompany with fresh fruit or a side salad of mixed greens.

Lean meats, whole grains, vibrant veggies, healthy fats, and delectable seasonings abound in these nutritious meal ideas, offering a mix of nutrients for satiety, energy, and general well-being. For tasty and nourishing meals,

modify the recipes according to your dietary requirements and tastes.

Desserts and Snacks to Maintain Blood Sugar Balance

Desserts and snacks can provide a regulated blood sugar level while still being enjoyable. The following are some suggestions for low-GI foods, fiber, healthy fats, and nutrient-dense snacks and desserts:

Ideas for Healthful Snacks:

Greek Yogurt Concession:

Top Greek yogurt with chopped nuts or seeds (almonds, walnuts, or chia seeds), fresh berries (strawberries, blueberries, or raspberries), a drizzle of honey, or a dash of cinnamon. When it comes to sugar content, Greek yogurt is less than flavored yogurt and more in protein.

Sticks of vegetables with hummus:

Dip celery sticks, bell pepper strips, carrot sticks, and cucumber slices into store-bought or homemade hummus. Hummus' protein and vegetables' fiber work together to stabilize blood sugar.

Apple Slices with Almond Butter: For a filling and crispy snack, spread almond butter on apple slices. A balanced energy boost is provided by the fiber in apples and the healthy fats in almond butter, which don't quickly raise blood sugar levels.

Hard-Boiled Eggs: Packed full of protein, hard-boiled eggs are a quick and easy snack. For extra taste and nutrients, serve them with a side of cherry tomatoes or with a dash of salt and pepper.

Mixed Nuts and Seeds: For a crunchy and nutrient-dense snack, combine unsalted nuts (such as almonds, cashews, and pistachios) with seeds (like sunflower and pumpkin seeds).

Nuts and seeds are rich sources of healthy fats, fiber, and protein. Ideas for Healthful Desserts:

Berries with a Dark Chocolate Cover:

Fresh berries, like raspberries or strawberries, can be dipped into melted dark chocolate that has at least 70% cacao. Berries add natural sweetness

and fiber, while dark chocolate has less sugar and antioxidants.

Pudding with Chia Seeds:

Combine chia seeds, unsweetened almond or coconut milk, a small amount of vanilla extract, and a natural sweetener such as stevia or monk fruit to make a chia seed pudding. Place it in the refrigerator to thicken, and then garnish with chopped cinnamon or fresh fruit.

Apples Baked with Cinnamon:

After coring the apples, dust them with cinnamon. Bake till soft, then serve hot.

For added taste and texture, you may also mix in a dollop of Greek yogurt or a sprinkling of chopped nuts.

Spread Greek yogurt on a baking sheet covered with parchment paper to make frozen yogurt bark. Top with chopped almonds, seeds, unsweetened dried fruit, and a drizzle of melted dark chocolate. Freeze until solid, then break into pieces to enjoy a tasty and adaptable frozen dessert.

Avocado Chocolate Mousse: Until smooth and creamy, blend ripe avocado, cocoa powder, almond milk, vanilla extract, and a natural sweetener (such as honey or maple syrup). Let cool completely before serving for a rich, nutrient-dense dessert.

These treats and snacks have whole foods, good fats, and thoughtful amounts of natural sweeteners to help maintain blood sugar balance while satisfying cravings. Consume these sweets sparingly as part of a healthy, balanced diet.

CONCLUSION

Taking Control of Your Blood Sugar Balance to Empower You

By being proactive in understanding, managing, and optimizing your blood sugar levels, you may empower yourself through blood sugar balance. Here are some essential tactics and realizations to support you on your path to empowerment:

Knowledge and Consciousness:

When it comes to controlling blood sugar, information is power. Learn about blood sugar, including what it is, how it is measured, and the variables that affect it, including heredity, stress, physical activity, food, and drugs.

Learn how to analyze glucose monitoring data, such as fasting blood sugar, postprandial (after-meal) readings, and HbA1c levels. Gain an understanding of the distinctions between normal blood sugar levels, prediabetes, and diabetes.

Optimal Eating Practices:

Make an effort to eat a balanced diet rich in a range of nutrient-dense foods, including whole grains, fruits, vegetables, lean meats, and healthy fats.

Aim for attentive eating, portion control, and regular meal timing. To assist regulate blood sugar levels and prevent sharp spikes and crashes, choose foods with a lower glycemic index.

Eat fewer processed foods, sugar-filled beverages, refined carbohydrates, and high-fat foods as these can hurt blood sugar regulation.

Frequent Exercise:

Make regular exercise a part of your routine; it can help lower blood sugar, increase insulin sensitivity, and promote general health.

As advised by health guidelines, choose enjoyable activities like walking, cycling, swimming, dancing, or strength training, and try to get at least 150 minutes of moderate-intensity activity per week.

Stress management: Insulin resistance and high blood sugar levels can both be caused by prolonged stress. Engage in stress-relieving activities such as gradual muscle relaxation, yoga, meditation, deep breathing, mindfulness, and enjoyable hobbies.

Make getting enough sleep and engaging in restorative activities a priority to help your body manage stress hormones and enhance general well-being.

Frequent Monitoring and Tracking: To monitor your blood sugar levels and identify trends over time, use continuous glucose monitoring (CGM) systems, blood glucose monitoring devices, or routine lab testing.

To track your food intake, exercise, medication use, stress levels, and other pertinent aspects that may affect your blood sugar control, utilize digital tools or keep a notebook. You can use this information to spot trends and make well-informed decisions regarding your health.

Collaboration and Adherence to Medication:

If your doctor has recommended medicine to control your blood sugar, take it as instructed and report any side effects or concerns right away.

Together with your medical team—which could consist of physicians, nurses, dietitians, pharmacists, and other experts—create a customized treatment plan that takes into account your particular requirements, objectives, and preferences.

Support and Modifications to Lifestyle:

Think about adopting healthier lifestyle choices that promote blood sugar balance, such as giving up drinking and smoking, controlling long-term health issues like high blood pressure or cholesterol, and keeping a healthy weight.

Seek out assistance from loved ones, friends, online forums, support groups, and medical experts. They may provide resources, advice, and encouragement to help you stay motivated and dedicated to your blood sugar control objectives.

Blood sugar balancing is a journey that may empower you, but it takes perseverance, self-awareness, and commitment. You may take charge of your blood sugar levels and enhance your general quality of life by being proactive about your health, making wise decisions, and asking for help when you need it. Keep in mind that gradual, tiny changes over time can result in big gains, and acknowledge your accomplishments as you go.